Praise for]
Chinese Sham

"Zhongxian Wu's latest book, *Chinese Shamanic Cosmic Orbit Qigong*, successfully continues his previous explorations of the highly secret shamanic tradition of self-cultivation as practiced on Mt. Emei in Sichuan. He provides a comprehensive and very accessible introduction to the main concepts and principles, then outlines 12 distinct exercises that tend to focus on the internal guiding and activation of Qi, supported by hand and arm movements as well as mental visualizations and specific breathing patterns. The exercises can be done one by one or in an integrated sequence. They offer a potent introduction to Daoist meditation and open a unique access to our internal energies. A great book for beginners and advanced practitioners alike."

—*Livia Kohn, Ph.D., Professor Emerita of Religion and East Asian Studies, Boston University*

by the same author

The 12 Chinese Animals
Create Harmony in Your Daily Life Through
Ancient Chinese Wisdom
ISBN 978 1 84819 031 3

Hidden Immortal Lineage Taiji Qigong
The Mother Form
DVD
ISBN 978 1 84819 040 5

Seeking the Spirit of The Book of Change
8 Days to Mastering a Shamanic Yijing (I Ching)
Prediction System
Foreword by Daniel Reid
ISBN 978 1 84819 020 7

Vital Breath of the Dao
Chinese Shamanic Tiger Qigong—Laohu Gong
Foreword by Chungliang Al Huang
ISBN 978 1 84819 000 9

Chinese Shamanic Cosmic Orbit Qigong

Esoteric Talismans, Mantras, and Mudras in Healing and Inner Cultivation

Master Zhongxian Wu

SINGING
DRAGON

LONDON AND PHILADELPHIA

First published in 2011
by Singing Dragon
an imprint of Jessica Kingsley Publishers
116 Pentonville Road
London N1 9JB, UK
and
400 Market Street, Suite 400
Philadelphia, PA 19106, USA

www.singingdragon.com

Library of Congress Cataloging in Publication Data
A CIP catalog record for this book is available from the Library of Congress

British Library Cataloguing in Publication Data
A CIP catalogue record for this book is available from the British Library

ISBN 978 1 84819 056 6

Printed and bound in the United States

This book is dedicated to
Ancient Chinese Wu 巫 *Traditions*
and Master Yu Wencai 于文才

Contents

Acknowledgments

In 2001, I decided to share my traditions with the Western audience and accordingly, planned to write a series of books on Chinese wisdom written in English. I see this book as an unforeseen special bonus! In my tradition, *Wu* 巫 (Chinese Shamanic) Cosmic Orbit Qigong is one of the most secret practices, and I originally did not intend to write about it. I knew that it would take great skill to effectively relay the inner nuances of this powerful and empowering form to any student. Additionally, when it comes to the complete transmission of knowledge to students, I am well aware that words alone will never suffice. A decade has now passed. Inspired by years of enthusiasm from my students and from other Qigong practitioners, I now realize that words can indeed rouse the spirit, be motivation for our inner cultivation practice, and help awaken our consciousness. Through this book, I hope to encourage people to seek out teachers who are upholding traditional Chinese wisdom cultivation techniques.

I would like to thank Deidre Orceyre—the first to encourage me to write about this form (and who created the earliest version of the Quick Review Chart found in Appendix I), and all those who have given me feedback along the way and supported my teaching—both live and in written form.

I would like to express my deepest gratitude to the spirit of *Wu* lineage and to my masters. They are the unlimited source of wisdom that guides my writing.

I extend many thanks to Jessica Kingsley and her Singing Dragon for her continued support of my work.

I also have great appreciation for Helena Ström Taylor. It is through her creative talent that my calligraphy and drawings are transformed into book-ready form.

And, of course, I offer special acknowledgment to my precious wife, Karin Elizabeth Taylor Wu, for her outstanding skills as my Editor-in-Chief, and for her gentle spirit of love, care, and support in our daily life together.

Harmonious Qi,

Zhongxian Wu
December 2, 2010

CHINESE SHAMANIC QIGONG

1. The Shamanic Root of Qigong 气功

When I was a child in China, I was curious about the way that the local *Wu* 巫 (Chinese shaman) would give treatments to patients. How could an acupuncture needle release the pain when the *Wu* placed it in a suffering patient's body? How could chanting, meditation, and use of talismans help patients recover from illness? Although I gathered more knowledge about the principles of Chinese medicine as I grew up, I did not get answers to my questions during my childhood. Ever inquisitive, I sought the answer to more questions: What are meridians? What are acupuncture points? Where did this knowledge come from? How did this intricately layered system of medicine develop? Through decades of dedicated Qigong and self-cultivation practices, I gradually found the answers to these questions. As my practice of ancient Chinese wisdom techniques deepened, I began to understand that ancient *Wu* 巫 (Chinese shamanism) is the root of all Chinese culture.

By Chinese shamanic definition, the Universe is the union of time and space. Time is specifically defined as past, present, and future, while space is described as above, below, front, back, left, and right. Ancient *Wu* 巫 (shamans) applied these concepts to their bodies, understanding their bodies to be their stable center and a "high-tech" vehicle of communication with the energies of time and space.

Profoundly connected with nature, ancient *Wu* 巫 (shamans) recognized that the life force of nature is composed of the interaction of one Yin (light energy), one Yang (heavy energy), and the expression of that duality throughout the Universe. Heaven represents the Yang component of this dichotomy whereas Earth represents the Yin aspect. It is the balanced union of these heavenly Yang and earthly Yin energies that results in the state of oneness, or "Universe," where peace and harmony can be experienced in a palpable way; for example, when communities are at peace with one another, the farmers are wholistically yielding a bountiful crop, and individuals are living sustainable, healthy, and happy lives. Likewise, imbalances in these energies can result in disharmony in the world, which can manifest as warfare, famine, destruction of ecosystems, natural disasters, and epidemic diseases.

As a vital part of this dynamic universe, human beings are also subject to the effects of these energies. In ancient China, shamans were respected as sages and enlightened beings who understood the way of nature and how it related to human beings. Ancient Chinese shamans considered human beings to be the precious treasure residing between heaven and earth. How, then, does one protect this precious life? Through study and observation of the Universal way, the ancient Chinese sages realized that achieving harmony in the body is possible when a person follows the balancing principles of the Universe in everyday living. With living in harmony as the ultimate goal, the ancient shamans created an ancient life science system designed to keep the physical body, the mind, and the spirit healthy. Today, we know this ancient life science system as Qigong 气功.

2. Choose a Beneficial Qigong 气功 Form

The term Qigong is made with two Chinese characters: Qi 气 and Gong 功. In English, Qi translates conceptually as vital energy, vital force, or vital breath, while Gong translates as working hard in the correct way. In general, Qigong 气功 means Qi cultivation. Any movements, postures or activity done in a conscious relationship with Qi can be called Qigong. There are many Qigong practices: sitting meditation, movement (including Taijiquan and other martial arts), breath work, visualization, regulation of mental focus and emotions, mudra, and mantra. The proper use of herbal medicines and food choices can also be considered a practice of Qigong. When done mindfully, cultivation of the arts, such as calligraphy and music, are also Qigong. In sum, Qigong is anything that facilitates the development of a deeper relationship with Qi and consciousness, which in turn helps the practitioner to understand the laws of the Universe and how they influence his or her life. If you are not yet aware of the Qi flowing through and around your body, you can cultivate this consciousness through a correct traditional Qigong practice and develop a better understanding of your internal and external Qi network. In its true form, Qigong is a practice for cultivating wisdom and a direct method for moving into *Tian Ren He Yi* 天人合一 (the union of nature and human being).

In our modern age, there are now literally thousands of Qigong forms in existence. Increasingly more people, both Eastern and Western, are interested in Qigong because of the great benefits gained from a regular practice. It is easy to find a Qigong book or DVD to start you on this journey. However, please be aware that the layers of wisdom and knowledge that come through your Qigong practice can simply not be learned through books and DVDs alone. Qigong is a way of cultivating knowledge and a method of practice that should be learned through correct and careful guidance and through personal experience. You will feel it is easier to merge the principles of your Qigong practice into your life and to feel its powerful effects if you have the support of an experienced teacher to guide you. People often ask me what kind of Qigong form will be suitable for them. I always suggest that they choose a traditional style of Qigong, one with deep cultural roots that has proven to be authentic over centuries of practice. Authenticity is one of the most important standards for beginning Qigong practitioners to be aware of when choosing a Qigong style.

3. Wu 巫 (Chinese Shamanic) Cosmic Orbit Qigong

Wu (Chinese Shamanic) Cosmic Orbit Qigong comes from *Emei Zhengong* 峨嵋真功 (Mt. Emei Sage Style Qigong),* which focuses on connecting to the universal energies of Heaven, Earth, and Humanity for the purpose of cultivating internal Qi circulation and attaining enlightenment. Mt. Emei Sage Style Qigong combines the traditions of ancient *Wu* (shamanism), Confucianism, Daoism, Classical Chinese Medicine, and the martial arts. The elements of this lineage are rooted in the ancient world of Chinese shamanism, which itself is the very source of all the classical Chinese traditions. The theoretical foundation of Mt. Emei Sage Style Qigong

---

* If you are interested in learning the detailed lineage history of Mt. Emei Sage Style Qigong (*Emei Zhengong*) please read my book *Vital Breath of the Dao—Chinese Shamanic Tiger Qigong (Laohu Gong)*, also published by Singing Dragon.

is embedded in *Yijing* (*I Ching*) science and the principles of Classical Chinese Medicine. This style has strong *Fulu* 符籙 practice, which holds some rituals and secret methods that are similar to those in the *Wu* (Chinese shamanic) and Daoist *Fulu* tradition. The Chinese character *Fu* means symbol, omen, talisman, in alignment with, or in accord with. *Lu* refers to the book of prophesy, incantation, or an energetic amulet (a charm to ward off evil or to create harmonious Qi). Because of its ancient Chinese shamanic ritual practices, the *Fulu* school is the core spirit of the *Wu* (Chinese shamanic school). As is common to practices that have been passed down through ancient shamanic Qigong lineages, Mt. Emei Sage Style Qigong includes the use of *Jue* 訣 (mantras), *Yin* 印 (mudras), visualizations, and conscious connection to the "Qi field" of the lineage, in addition to the more commonly known aspects of breath, movement, stillness, and connection to universal energies that are found in all traditional styles of Qigong.

Three essential practices of Chinese Shamanic Qigong are the *Fu* 符 (talismans), *Jue* 訣 (mantras), and *Yin* 印 (mudras). Talisman, mudra, and mantra are specific rituals common to ancient shamanism. In Mt. Emei Sage Style Qigong, we still preserve and utilize many special talismans, mantras, and mudras as specific techniques for cultivation and healing/ self-healing. *Fu* (talismans) are Qi (vital life energy) energized diagrams, symbols, or Chinese characters used to channel vital energy in order to create a harmonious Qi field for healing or living. *Jue* (mantras) are special syllables, spells, or sounds used to resonate with Universal Qi and circulate the Qi within the energy network through the vibrations created by the voice. *Yin* (mudras) are ancient hand positions used to connect with universal energies and act as a vehicle to access the ancient wisdom of the Universe that is bound within the body. *Wu* (Chinese Shamanic) Cosmic Orbit Qigong combines *Fu* (talismans), *Jue* (mantras), and *Yin* (mudras) with each movement.

Wu (Chinese Shamanic) Orbit Qigong is a time-honored, esoteric style of *Zhoutian* 周天 (Cosmic Orbit) Qigong practice. In Chinese, *Zhou* means cycle, circular, perfect, complete, and rotate; *Tian* means sky, heaven, and universe; together, the original meaning of *Zhoutian* describes the complete circle as made by the Earth's daily rotation around its axis. Commonly, *Zhoutian* translates as cosmic orbit. Through inner cultivation practices, ancient shamans discovered that the energetic patterns of human beings mirror those of the Universe. If the same patterns are reproduced in all levels of the cosmos, from the largest, macrocosmic (Universal level) scale to the smallest, microcosmic (e.g. living organisms and the cells, organelles and particles within them) scale, they deduced that the flow of Qi in the body is just like the ceaseless rotation of the sun, moon, and stars. Therefore, in Qigong terminology, *Zhoutian* also refers to the specific pattern of Qi circulation in the body. The fundamental concept of balance in Chinese wisdom traditions holds that you will maintain health and experience well-being if Qi is free flowing in your body.

In 1996, a group of Chinese medicine students from the West came to China to study with me. To my knowledge, this was the first opportunity for anyone from the Western world to learn the practice of the shamanic style *Zhoutian* (cosmic orbit) Qigong. In 2001, I left China and moved to the United States. Over the years, I have held numerous workshops on this form, and have had feedback from many of my students that this form is simple, powerful, and easy to learn. In my experience, practitioners gain tremendous cumulative benefits through daily practice of this Shamanic Orbit Qigong. Many of my students have asked that I write about the form in order to help them further understand the form in their daily home practice. In 2003, I prepared a booklet about Shamanic Orbit

Qigong to help support these Qigong friends in their practice. Now, seven years later, I feel it is time to expand upon my earlier writings and share this authentic practice, spirit intact, with the general public. This book illustrates the details of the Shamanic Orbit Qigong practice, including talismans, mantras, mudras, movements, visualizations, and therapeutic benefits. In Appendix I, you will find a Quick Review Chart of the form. I hope you will enjoy the Mt. Emei Sage Style Shamanic Cosmic Orbit Qigong. In terms of your physical and emotional health and your spiritual evolution, you will be well rewarded if you are able to find an experienced teacher to guide you through the intricacies of the practice.

.

THE
PRACTICE

1

Yang Sheng Yuan Hai

陽生元海

Generating Your Vitality

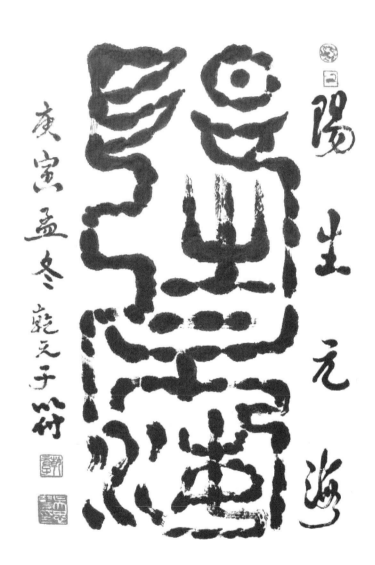

陽生元海

庚寅孟冬範无子以符

Meaning

As I discussed in my book, *Vital Breath of the Dao—Chinese Shamanic Tiger Qigong (Laohu Gong)*, the name of a Qigong form contains the essence and spirit of the form. Gaining an appreciation of the name of a form or movement will help us master our Qigong practice. At the beginning of each chapter of this section of the book, I will first interpret the name of the movement in order to facilitate bringing you into a deep understanding and experience of the practice.

In this movement, **Yang** 陽 means high brightness, which refers to the sun. The sun symbolizes the wisdom and spirit of the body in Chinese spiritual cultivation practices. It is a symbol for vital energy, brightness, activity, openness, vigor, and power. **Sheng** 生 means vitality, new life, life force, creation, generation, create, and make. **Yuan** 元 means origin, source, and spring. **Hai** 海 means great lake, sea, and ocean. In Chinese *Wu* 巫 (shamanic) traditions, we believe that all life originates from water. We understand that everyone's life source comes from the "great water" of the body, which is located in the lower abdomen in an area we call *Yuanhai* 元海—the original ocean of your life source.

Yang Sheng Yuan Hai is the foundation of your Qigong practice. It is a way to generate your new life energy, which is known as the *Yang* 陽 or *Yangqi* 陽炁 in traditional internal alchemy practices and other methods of Chinese inner cultivation techniques.

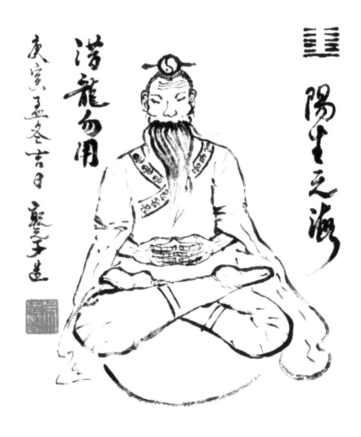

Figure 1. Generating Your Vitality Posture

Movement

Straighten your back so that it feels as solid as a mountain. Lift your perineum (the small area between your sexual organs and your anus) to seal the *Dihu* 地戶. *Dihu*, or Earthly Door, is an acupuncture point known as "*Huiyin* 會陰" (CV1), which is located in your perineum. Pull your lower abdomen in. To open your chest, bring your shoulders slightly back and down. Straighten your neck and keep your head upright. Imagine the top of your head is touching heaven with *Tianmen* 天門 open. *Tianmen*, also known as Heavenly Gate, is the acupuncture point called "*Baihui* 百會" (GV20), which is located on the top of your head. Place the tip of your tongue on the tooth ridge behind your upper teeth. Keep your teeth and mouth closed. With shoulders down, arms relaxed, and armpits slightly open, make the ***Chunyangyin*** 純陽印—Pure Yang Mudra—over the lower *Dantian* 丹田 (Figure 1). Your *Dantian* (*Dan* means elixir, which symbolizes the eternal life source, and *tian* means field) is your elixir field, and is located in your lower belly.

To make the Pure Yang Mudra, bring your thumbs, middle fingers and little fingers together. Straighten the second and fourth fingers. This Chinese name of *Chunyangyin* 純陽印 carries multiple layers of meaning and also contains its intentions. According to the second-century dictionary, *Analyzing Simple Lines and Explaining Complex Graphs* (*Shuowen Jiezi* 说文解字), the original meaning of *Chun* 純 is silk. The symbolic meaning of silk is white, pure, and link or connection. Therefore, the character *Chun* exemplifies pure, purity, or purifying connection. *Yang* 陽 also contains many layers of meaning, including sun, heaven, and brightness. *Yang* has a positional meaning as well, and can be used to reference the area south of a hill or north of a river, which are the areas that typically get more sunshine and therefore have more life energy. *Yin* 印 conveys the meaning of an official seal. In the terminology of the Chinese shamanic or Daoist traditions, *Yin* also means mudra. Put together, these three terms make *Chunyangyin*, which tells us that the function of this mudra is to help the practitioner connect with Universal Qi 炁, the vital energy of the Universe. This practice purifies the body and transforms the practitioner's energy into pure Yang energy.

Visualization

Relax your eyelids and turn your eyesight within, bringing it back to your body. Look within, listen within, and visualize the Qi state, in which your whole body is soaking in the sunlight. Open all the pores of your skin, and allow the Universal Qi, like sunlight, to flow into your body through your skin. Feel your body merging with the light. Imagine both hands are holding a fireball or golden-red sun in your lower *Dantian*.

Breathing

Adjust your breathing to be slow, smooth, deep, and even. Your breath should be soundless. In Chinese, *mi mi mian mian* 密密綿綿 means breathing that is soft and unbroken like cotton or silk. Gather the Universal Qi into your body through all the pores of your skin as your inhale. As you exhale, merge the Qi with the fireball or golden-red sun that you are imagining in your lower belly. Observe your body and inner landscape through your breath. After a few minutes of this breathing practice, sound the Mantra **Heng** 哼 (pronounced "Hung" and meaning sacrificial offering) nine times to strengthen your Yang Qi or life force.

Benefit

This posture, especially when combined with the mudra, will help increase your energy. Your five fingers are connected with the *Wuxing* 五行, or five phases, which are the very essence of classical Chinese philosophy. The five phases (commonly referred to as five "elements") are Water, Wood, Fire, Earth, and Metal. They are the fundamental components of everything in the Universe, which, as we discussed in the introduction, includes all temporal and spatial concepts.

Your body, of course, is also made up of these fundamental components. In Chinese medicine, the five fingers on your hand are considered *Wai Wuxing* 外五行 (external five phases or five elements), and they correspond to the *Nei Wuxing* 內五行 (internal five phases or elements), which define the five organ systems of your body. For example, the first finger (i.e. the little finger) connects with your kidneys and everything in the Universe represented by the Water element. The second finger, the ring finger, is a link between your liver and the Wood element. The middle finger, number three, is related to your heart and the Fire element. Your fourth finger is your index finger, and it is associated with your lungs and the Metal element. Finally, your thumb, the fifth finger, carries a relationship with your spleen and the Earth element. In the numerology of the *Yijing* 易經, 1, 2, 3, 4, and 5 are known as the creation numbers. These five numbers are also called the five elements' numbers. According to *Yijing Yinyang* 陰陽 principle, all of the even numbers have *Yin* 陰 qualities whereas all the odd numbers are *Yang* 陽 in nature. Yin represents gentle, soft, hidden, unclear, dark, moon, feminine, mother, and earth while Yang represents tough, hard, flaunt, clear, bright, sun, masculine, father, and heaven.

The Pure Yang Mudra is made with fingers 1, 3, and 5. Added together, 1 + 3 + 5 = 9. The number 9 is the highest Yang number in the five elements number system. In the *Yijing*, the number nine is the original depiction of the concept of Yang. 2 + 4 = 6 when added together. Six is the purest and highest Yin number in the five elements number system. In the *Yijing*, the number six was the original depiction of the concept of Yin. If you are interested in *Yijing* numerology, you can find some more details in my earlier book, *Seeking the Spirit of The Book of Change—8 Days to Mastering a Shamanic Yijing (I Ching) System*, also published by Singing Dragon.

By connecting the little fingers, middle fingers and thumbs, you can connect to, adjust, and improve your body's Yang energy. One important thing to remember is that Yin always nourishes Yang. Therefore, when holding this mudra, be sure to keep the second and fourth fingers open so that you connect with all the energy (Yin and Yang) in the Universe. When you open Yin and connect with the Universe, you nourish your whole body. The ring finger and index finger are connected with soul energy, a special spiritual form of Qi. What is this soul energy? We call it the *Hun* 魂 and *Po* 魄. From a Chinese medicine perspective, the liver stores *Hun* and the lung stores *Po*. Although the *Hun* and *Po* are complex concepts with several meanings, we can simplify those concepts here and understand that within a person's body, *Hun* is Yang spiritual energy and *Po* is Yin spiritual energy. These energies are eternal. When a person dies, *Hun* rises into the heaven and *Po* sinks into the earth.

The pictograms for *Hun* and *Po* can also help us understand this. The character *Hun* is made up of two radicals. On the left, we see the radical for cloud 云, and on the right we see the character, *Gui* 鬼. *Gui* means ghost, and according to *Analyzing Simple Lines and Explaining Complex Graphs (Shuowen Jiezi* 说文解字), it means "a person returning back to her/his origins." The character *Po* features the radical *Bai* 白 on the left and the same *Gui* component on the right. *Bai* means white, and one of its symbolic meanings is metal. The tendency of clouds is to ascend and stay in the sky while the tendency of metal is to descend and bury itself in the earth. *Hun* is Yang energy related to the heavens and *Po* is Yin energy related to the earth. In Chinese internal alchemy, *Hun* is manifested in the Sun and *Po* is manifested in the Moon. The Sun and the Moon present the clearest picture of Yang and Yin. Ancient Chinese sages understood the *Dao* 道 (the Universal or Eternal Way) through careful and diligent observation of the opposite nature of the Sun and the Moon. The ring finger and index fingers in the Pure Yang Mudra also represent the Sun (*Hun*) and the Moon (*Po*). The Sun and the Moon have never stopped their rotation and their revolution. This is the eternal way of the Universe. When we follow the Universal Way, we emulate this pattern through our commitment to our daily cultivation practices.

Yang Sheng Yuan Hai will help you connect to your infinite life source and will enhance your vitality.

2

Xin Di Kuan Rong
心地寬容

Connecting with the Earth

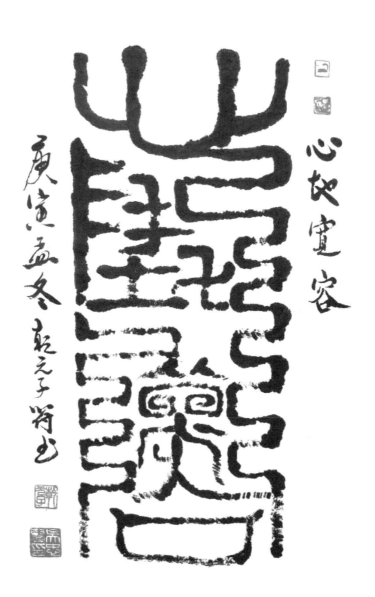

心地寬容

庚寅孟冬
乾元子肖山

Meaning

Xin 心 means heart and mind. *Di* 地 means earth, land, and field. *Kuang* 寬 means wide, expand, and open. *Rong* 容 means contain, hold, and embrace. In Chinese wisdom traditions, we hold that one of the most important functions of the heart is that of fertile soil, a place where the seeds of our thoughts and attitudes are sown. Just as different seeds planted in the earth grow into a wide variety of plants, the seeds of new thoughts and attitudes that are planted in our hearts will grow into plants that yield various fruits in our lives. Ancient wisdom teaches us that positive thoughts or attitudes will bring positive conditions into our lives, whereas negative thoughts or attitudes will lead us to experience more negative circumstances.

During inner cultivation practices, it is important to cultivate your *Xindi* 心地, the heart/mind with the qualities of the Earth—open, straightforward, greatness, gentleness, compassionate, and forgiving. The Earth gives birth to Ten Thousand Things, nourishing them without asking for reward. By living in accordance with this function of the Earth, you will develop an expansive, open heart that will be able to smooth all manner of suffering in your life. Traditionally, purifying your heart is one of the most important steps in starting your inner cultivation practices, just as when farmers clear weeds from their fields before sowing their seeds. If you want to have healthy physical and spiritual growth, clear out your mental and spiritual "weeds," and allow your breath to cleanse negative thoughts, attitudes, and all manner of mental and emotional stagnation.

Xin Di Kuan Rong is a way to purify your heart and learn to "let it be." It is also a powerful way to heal any type of health issues that are related to mental, emotional, and spiritual imbalances.

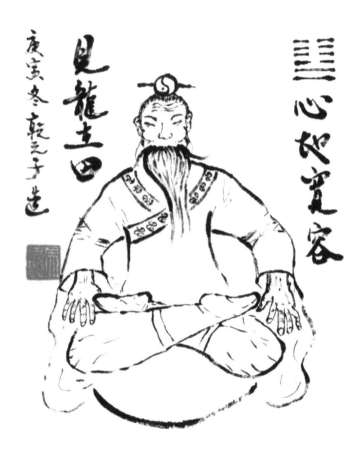

Figure 2. Connecting with the Earth Posture

Movement

Release the mudra from the previous posture by slowly opening your arms and turning the wrists so that your palms face earth and your forearms are parallel to the ground. End with your fingertips pointing forward and your forearms parallel to each other. This position is *Xindiyin* 心地印—Heart Earth Mudra (Figure 2). Practicing this mudra will help your heart connect with the gracious qualities of Mother Earth, and help release any stagnating patterns in your mental–emotional state.

Visualization

Imagine the fingers and the *Laogong* 勞宮 connecting with the earth. The *Laogong* are acupuncture points located at the center of your palms (also known as "Palace of Weariness" or PC8) that connect to your pericardium (the heart protector) and your heart. Feel your hands and your entire body merging into the earth with golden yellow Qi.

Breathing

Deeply inhale while opening your hands and moving into *Xindiyin*. Hold the posture while keeping your breath slow, smooth, deep, and even. Sound the Mantra **Hu** 呼 five times. *Hu* (pronounced "hoo") means blow off or clear out. Practicing this mantra can help release your stress and ease your heart/mind.

Benefit

In Traditional Chinese Medicine, there are ten acupuncture points located at the tips of each of your fingers. These special points, named *Shixuan* 十宣, act as the gateways between the microcosm (your body) and the macrocosm (the Universe). *Shi* means ten. *Xuan* means declare, transmit, express, understand, clear, all around, link up, and communicate. These ten points are some of most sensitive points in the body and thus are readily used to receive and transmit Qi. Over time, practicing this posture will help you open your *Shixuan* (ten emitting points) at the ten finger tips and your *Laogong*, thus strengthening your ability to connect with Earthly Qi. Through this connection, you will nurture your ability to forgive, to develop true compassion for yourself and others, and to connect with your pure heart.

With respect to your physical body, this practice will also help you balance your blood pressure, strengthen the function of your circulation systems (including Qi, blood, and lymph), and improve the physiological function of your heart and digestive system.

3

Xiu Zhuan Qian Kun
袖轉乾坤

Communicating with the Heavens

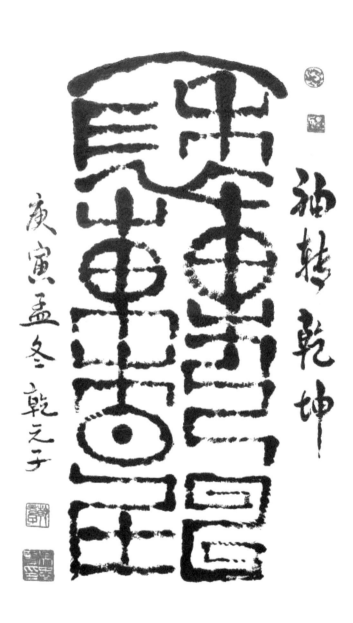

袖转乾坤

庚寅孟冬 乾之子

Meaning

The meaning of **Xiu** 袖 is sleeve. **Zhuang** 轉 means turn, rotate, and switch. **Qian** 乾, the name of a trigram and a hexagram in the *Yijing*, has an original meaning of rising Qi 氣 or energy. According to ancient Chinese cosmology, the ascending Qi formed Heaven, and *Qian* therefore also represents Heaven. By Heaven we do not simply mean Heaven or sky, but all functions of the Universe, including the movements of the planets and stars. The movement of the cosmos is absolutely present and is in constant motion. This is the energetic meaning of *Qian*. We use *Qian* to represent anything that has a strong uplifting and unwavering spirit or energetic quality. *Qian* is that which draws upward and perseveres, just like the planets in the sky above keep their rotation and never stop running. **Kun** 坤 is also the name of a trigram and a hexagram in the *Yijing*. It represents the Earth quality of openness, greatness, and carrying everything. Like the mother, the Earth holds everything. The Chinese character *Kun* is made by the left radical *Tu* 土, which means earth, soil, clay, and mud, and the right radical *Shen* 申, which means stretch, brightening, or spirit. Therefore, *Kun* symbolizes the Nature spirits that are hidden within the Earth. Earth does not show off, yet it holds, carries, and supports all beings. When put together, *Qiankun* 乾坤 is one of the names for the Universe. Symbolically, it represents the role of karma or destiny in our cultivation practice. We have an expression, "the Universe is within my hand," which means that we are able to change the trajectory of our lives and our destiny through concentrated efforts. In China, our clothes traditionally have very long sleeves. We often keep our hands hidden within these sleeves during our Qi cultivation practices so that no one will be able to see the secrets of our hand movements. *Xiu Zhuang Qian Kun*, or turning the Universe with your hands (sleeves), is a

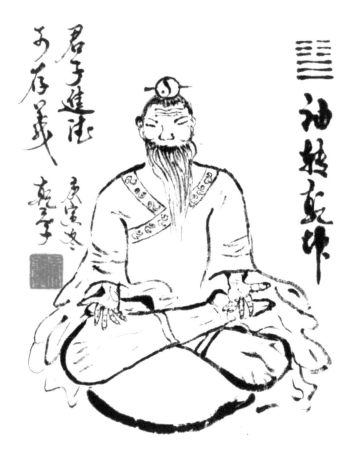

Figure 3. Communicating with the Heavens Posture

practice that will help you improve your life and your destiny, allowing you to live up to your greatest potential, in health and in harmony.

Movement

From the previous posture, continue opening your arms while rotating the fingers downwards, one by one (starting with the little fingers), and then your wrists so that palms are facing upwards. Feel that you are gathering the Universal Qi. While rotating, you are also moving your arms so that your hands end up slightly behind you. Keeping your wrists bent, palms and fingers facing upward, fold in your arms and bring your hands upwards towards your armpits. End with your fingers outstretched and palms facing heaven (at about waist level) in *Qiankunyin* 乾坤印—Heaven Earth Mudra. Your elbows are once again bent so that your forearms are parallel with the earth (Figure 3). In Chinese wisdom traditions, we consider the palm to hold Yin energy, signifying the Earthly aspects of your body, while the back of your hand contains the Yang energy and represents the Heavenly aspects of your body. The cyclical flow of Heavenly Qi (rain) and Earthly Qi (clouds) generates the harmony of nature. Similar to this natural pattern, practice *Qiankunyin* to create a free flow of your Yin and Yang energies and facilitate balance in your life.

Visualization

Imagine your fingers extend far away, and that you are collecting the Qi while rotating your fingers and wrists. Visualize that your hands are full of the lights from heaven as you hold the posture.

Breathing

Take a deep breath as you open your arms and rotate your fingers. Exhale slowly as you outstretch your fingers. Continue to breathe deeply and soundlessly as in previous postures. Remember, you are not only breathing with your lungs, but also with your skin and with all the pores of your body. Feel the Qi merging with your body through all your pores as you inhale. Merge the Qi into *Dantian* (your lower abdomen) as you exhale. Sound the Mantra *Xu* 嘘 (pronounced "shhh") eight times. *Xu*, the sound of the liver, means emptiness. Using it will help release any stagnation in the function of your liver.

Benefit

As I mentioned before, your five fingers are connected to the five elements and with your five organ systems. Your little finger is related to the Water organ system (which includes your kidney and bladder), your ring finger is related to the Wood organ system (your liver and gallbladder), your middle finger is related to the Fire organ system (comprising of your heart and small intestines), your index finger is related to the Metal organ system (meaning your lung and large intestines), and finally, your thumb is related to the Earth organ system (which is made of up your spleen, pancreas, and stomach). In ancient Chinese shamanic healing systems, including Traditional Chinese Medicine, we believe that the entire body is an intricate, intercommunicating network of these five systems. With any kind of health issue, no matter if experienced in the physical, mental, or spiritual planes, we can always find the connection to suboptimal functioning somewhere within these five organ systems. The cumulative effect of practicing the rotation of your fingers in this movement will bring balance to your five organ systems, help you recover from any kind of illness, and allow you to live in a peaceful and harmonious state. By helping to open your ten emitting points, this movement will also increase your external Qi and healing power, strengthening your ability to do healing work on your self and with others.

4

Cheng Tong Dao Zhen

誠通道真

Resonating with the Dao

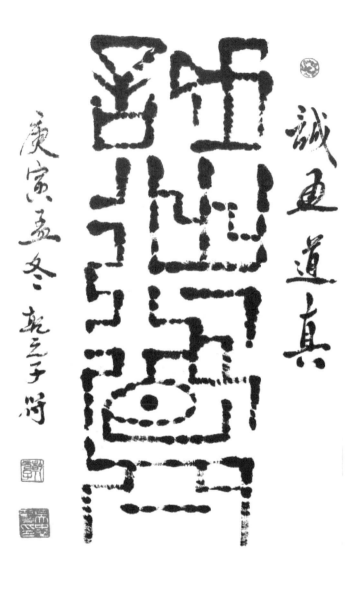

誠正道真

庚寅嘉冬 乾元子書

Meaning

Cheng 誠 means faith, trust, serious, sincere, honest, loyal, and faithful. *Tong* 通 means connect, communicate, and flow. *Dao* 道 means path, principle, and the Way—the way of nature and of the Universe. *Zhen* 真 means truth, reality, and immortality.

If you want to have the successful results of a dedicated inner cultivation practice, it is essential that you take the practice seriously. For instance, if you hold a meditation posture while watching television, you are not actually meditating and will not receive the same benefits as you would from holding the same posture in an earnest practice. Practicing Qigong is different from doing regular physical exercise; it directly engages mental, emotional, and spiritual processes. With a genuine practice, your heart will be able to resonate with the truth of your self, of nature, and of the great Dao. This will bring great benefits to your health and to your experience of daily life. Without *Cheng*, we will be not able to accomplish *Zhen*, a true experience and benefit of your inner cultivation practice.

In traditional Chinese culture, *Cheng* is the most crucial quality of our daily life and spiritual cultivation practice. In his writings, Confucius emphasized the many significant rewards of *Cheng*. *Cheng* is a way to connect with your almighty love, compassion, strength, and power; it is a way to awaken your consciousness and great wisdom; and it is a way to communicate with Heaven, Earth, and human beings— with great integrity.

Cheng Tong Dao Zhen is a way to help us deeply understand the reality of life, society, and nature. It is a profound way to help you connect with your heart.

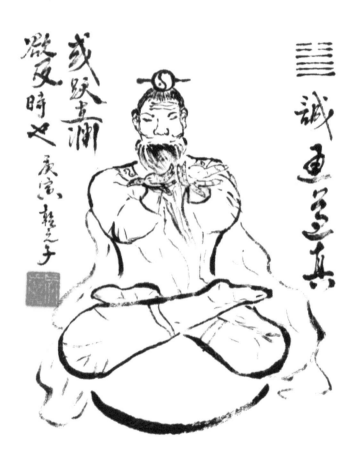

Figure 4. Resonating with the Dao Posture

Movement

From the previous posture, bring your arms straight out in front of you, at the level of your chest, with palms up. Make sure your thumb, index fingers and middle fingers are straight and pointing forward, and the ring fingers and little fingers bent and pointing towards heaven. This is the ***Daozhenyin*** 道真印—Daoist Reality Mudra (Figure 4). Practicing this mudra will help open your heart and cultivate true compassion, which is a path to the understanding reality of your life and the Dao.

Visualization

Imagine your fingertips are touching the ends of the Universe and penetrating Qi deep into the Universe. Feel your heart and entire body merging with the Universal Qi.

Breathing

While your hands are extending forward, exhale and sound the Mantra ***Hong*** 吽. Pronounced "hoang," *hong* translates as a powerful sound, like thunder, that connects with the Dao. This mantra is the voice of your heart, and using it will help your heart connect with your whole body and with nature.

Benefit

This practice will help you open your heart, revealing your great joy and compassion. It is also a way to strengthen the function of your physical heart and uplift your spirits.

Over the 20-plus years that I have been teaching Qigong, people have often asked how long they will need to practice a Qigong form before they will start to feel better. I always stress that the efficacy of your Qigong practice cannot be measured simply by the amount of time you have practiced, but rather is determined by the quality of your practice. In China, we have a saying—*bing dong san chi fei yi ri zhi han* 冰凍三尺非一日之寒 "Ice three feet deep does not form after a single day of freezing weather." In other words, reaping the harvest of your Qigong practice requires that you make a sincere and sustained effort to practice regularly. A Qigong form is easy to learn. The challenge most people face is having the strong determination to make their practice a part of their daily routine. It is frighteningly easy for people to find an excuse to skip a practice one day, then the next, and have it slip away. The key to maintaining your daily Qigong practice is to take it seriously, making a strong commitment to your self and your practice from deep within your unwavering heart/mind.

This movement will help you connect to your steadfast heart/mind, and through a daily practice will bring great strength to your mental, physical, and spiritual self.

5

San Cai He Yi

三才合一

Merging with the Universe

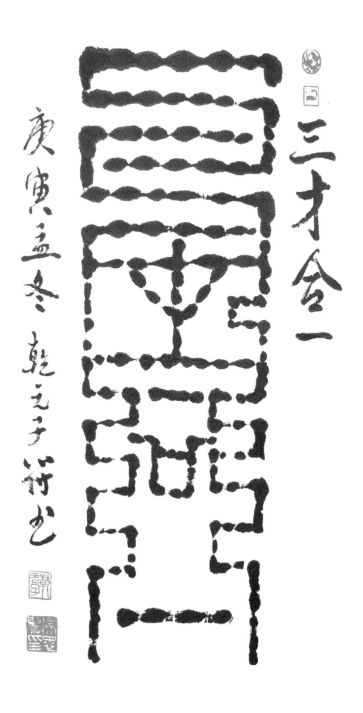

三才合一

庚寅孟冬 乾元子符書

Meaning

San 三 means the number three. In classical Chinese, three also means many or numerous. As you can see, it is made up of three horizontal lines which represent the three layers of the Universe—Heaven, Earth, and human being. In Chinese shamanic traditions, the number three is the creation number, it is the symbol of everything in the Universe, and of the Universe itself. *Cai* 才 means material and talent. *He* 合 means combine, merge, unite, union, unity, and harmony. *Yi* 一 means number one. It is a horizontal line (一) with two ends representing the combination of Yin and Yang. In Chinese numerology, the number one is also a symbol for unity and the Dao (the Way), representing stability and harmony.

In Chinese wisdom traditions, *Sancai* 三才, the trinity of the Universe, is a principle concept. "Three in one" is the pattern of nature—everything in nature is constructed of three layers or components. For instance, spatially, *Sancai* represents upper, middle, and lower. With reference to time, *Sancai* refers to past, present, and future. We talk about the sun, moon, and stars, and of fire, water, and wind being the *Sancai* in the sky and on the earth, respectively. *Jing* 精 (essence), Qi 氣 (vital energy), and *Shen* 神 (spirit) are the *Sancai* of the body. In Qigong practice, we will always work with three elements— posture, breath, and visualization. Laozi 老子 considered the union of this trinity to be the greatest accomplishment of nature, that which is responsible for all creation. Chapter 42 of the *Daodejing* 道德經 states:

道生一   The Dao gave birth to the One,

一生二   The One gave birth to the Two,

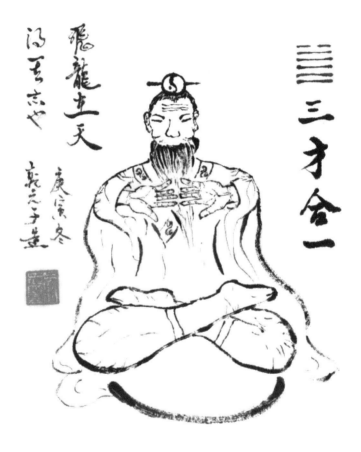

Figure 5. Merging with the Universe Posture

| 二生三 | The Two gave birth to the Three, |
| 三生万物 | And the Three gave birth to the 10,000 things. |

San Cai He Yi is a way to connect with the trinity of the Universe in order to strengthen and harmonize the three treasures of your body: your *Jing* (essence), Qi (vital energy), and *Shen* (spirit).

Movement

From the previous posture, bend your wrists towards you while rotating your fingers one by one (starting with the kidney finger). As you rotate your fingers, bend your elbows, and bring your hands closer to your body at the level of your middle *Dantian*, which is located at the center point between your nipples. Complete the rotation of your hands and wrists and turn your hands over so that your palms are now facing away from your middle *Dantian*. Your arms form an open circle in front of you with your elbows slightly bent and pointing towards each side. Your middle fingers are pointing towards each other, your little fingers point towards the sky and your thumbs are pointing towards the earth. This is the **Sancaiyin** 三才印—Trinity Mudra (Figure 5).

Visualization

Imagine your little fingers are touching heaven and merging with the Three Lights (the sun, moon, and stars). Visualize your thumbs connecting with the center of the earth and linking with the Three Sources—water, fire, and wind. Sense your *Laogong* connecting with the Universe in front of you, fusing in a harmonious union with your heart. In this mudra, your heart is represented by your middle fingers pointing horizontally towards each other. Feel your physical body melting into the Universal Qi field or into Universal light, and know that you are in a non-separate state.

Breathing

As with the previous movement, continue sounding the Mantra *Hong* 吽 as you exhale. Together, these two movements take place during one exhalation while using the same mantra.

Benefit

This practice can help facilitate a deeper opening of the heart, allowing you to sense and truly understand the union, or state of oneness, between human beings and nature. It is also a great way to improve your life force, your health, and your therapeutic power. You will be able to feel a dramatic increase in both your internal and external Qi after several weeks of practice. By communicating with the three heavenly lights and the three sources of Earthly energy, you will strengthen your own three treasures—*Jing*, Qi, and *Shen*.

6

Xiong Huai Wu Bian

胸懷無邊

Embracing Infinity

胸懷無邊

庚寅孟冬 乾之子 寫

Meaning

Xiong 胸 refers to the physical chest, which in Chinese tradition also represents the spiritual heart/mind. *Huai* 懷 means surround and embrace. *Wu* 無 means no, nothing, and empty. *Bian* 邊 means edge and boundary. *Wubian* means boundless, unlimited, vast, and infinity. During your inner cultivation practices, it is essential that you learn to let it be and refine your ability to detach. Please remember that detachment does not mean disconnection. Whether you feel great or badly about a situation or a person, if you can detach from it and let it go with love and compassion, your heart will be lightened. With time, you may experience the sensation of your heart expanding, and with it, the sky will feel higher, the ocean wider, and your life will feel boundless, overflowing with peace and harmony.

Your great heart (chest) is able to embrace the infinite quality of nature when it is full of love, joy, and compassion. Cultivating in this spirit will help you release the negative energies, such as jealousy, greed, anger, hatred, grief, longing, or desire, that may cause physical or mental challenges.

Xiong Huai Wu Bian illustrates that a key element for traditional Qigong practice is to cultivate your detachment, forgiveness, and big heart. It is a potent way to connect with the great Dao.

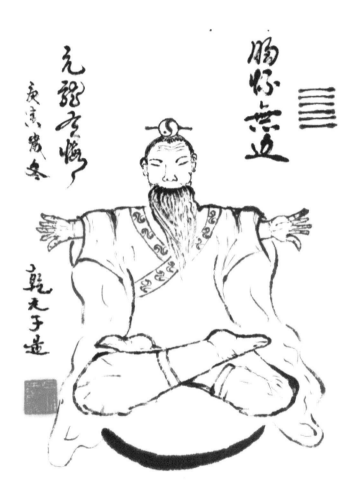

Figure 6. Embracing Infinity Posture

Movement

In a continuous movement from the previous posture, open your chest by moving your arms apart in an arc like fashion and drawing your shoulder blades together. Please make sure to keep stretching your fingers straight (with your little finger still stretching up towards heaven and thumb stretching down towards earth) and your elbows and your wrists slightly bent. At the end of the movement, your chest is open, your arms are stretched out to your sides, and your palms will be facing away from you in **Sixiangyin** 四象印—Four Spiritual Animals Mudra (Figure 6). In Chinese wisdom traditions, *Sixian* means four symbols. These specifically refer to the four spiritual animals—Green Dragon, White Tiger, Red Bird, and Black Warrior (a combination of turtle and snake). The four spiritual animals also represent the four directions—east, west, south, and north, and the four seasons—spring, autumn, summer, and winter. In traditional Qigong practice, the four spiritual animals are your spiritual guards.

Visualization

Imagine your *Laogong* touching the end of the Universe. As your chest opens, imagine the universal white or golden color Qi surrounding your body and feel your entire physical body is melting in the Qi field. Then visualize your spiritual guards—the Green Dragon on your left side, White Tiger on your right side, Red Bird in front of you, and the Black Warrior behind you.

Breathing

Take a deep breath, and with your exhale sound the Mantra **Ha** 哈 (pronounced "hah") while opening the chest and moving the hands outward. *Ha* means unite. Practicing this mantra will help you open your chest, enhance your lung Qi, improve your breathing function, and strengthen your ability to heal yourself and others.

Benefit

This practice will help enhance the function of your heart and lungs. The vibration of the Mantra *Ha* can be felt throughout the chest and entire body. It is one of the best practices to strengthen your lung Qi and will optimize functioning of your cardiovascular and respiratory systems. This practice is especially beneficial with regard to nurturing your ability to forgive and to expand your heart.

From my clinical experience, I find that many physical health problems are deeply rooted in the mental or spiritual levels. Please consider this if you experience difficulty achieving good healing results with yourself and/or with your clients. Cultivating the ability to "let it go" and to forgive yourself and others is an incredibly powerful healing modality. As Joseph Campbell states, "We must be willing to let go of the life we have planned, so as to accept the life that is waiting for us." You will be able to experience miraculous healing by mastering this practice.

7

Gui Gen Fu Ming

歸根復命

Returning to Your Root

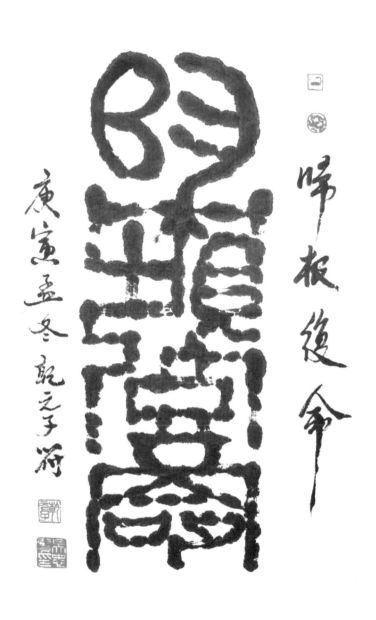

啼根復命

庚寅孟冬乾之子舒

Meaning

The original meaning of **Gui** 歸 is a bride or time of marriage. In Chinese tradition, a happy marriage establishes a peaceful and harmonious environment each time we return home, which helps create a lifetime of stability and success. The common meanings of *Gui* are secure, store, go back, and return. **Gen** 根 means root, source, and origin. The original meaning of **Fu** 復 is to walk back and forth, return, recover, and repeat. The original meaning of **Ming** 命 is order or command. According to ancient Chinese traditions, we believe that a person's life is commanded or ruled by the invisible universal law, the *Dao* 道. The Dao is the creative force behind all phenomena we interact with in our daily life. The phenomena, as it relates to your life, is known as *Ming*—karma or destiny.

In Chinese shamanic traditions, one of the central goals of inner cultivation is *Fuming* 復命—changing and improving your karma. In order to change your karma or destiny, you must first be able to understand it. In my opinion, the best way to understand your self and your karma is through your inner cultivation practice. Through your own strong commitment and effort, you will be able to recover your vital energy, regain your health, and feel peaceful and balanced in all aspects of your life. A way to *Fuming* is through the practice of *Guigen* 歸根—returning to your root, the root of your life source. You will find the infinite source of your own life energy and a deepening sense of peace as you bring your breath, your consciousness, and your spirit back to the place in your body in which your life energy originates.

Gui Gen Fu Ming is a way to change your life and karma, and is a way to find the source of peace and joy in your life.

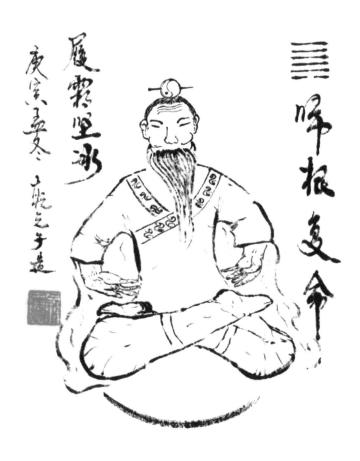

Figure 7. Returning to Your Root Posture

Movement

In a continuous movement from the previous posture, rotate your fingers, one by one (starting with the little finger) and bend your wrists so that your hands form a cup-like shape. Bring you hands around to your lower back. End the movement with the fingers and *Laogong* pointing toward the kidneys to make ***Jinguiyin*** 金龜印—Golden Turtle Mudra (Figure 7).

Turtles have the innate ability to find their way back to the place where they were born, regardless of how far they have traveled. Turtles are also capable of going for extended periods of time without taking in food as sustenance. According to *Wu* (Chinese shamanic) traditions, the Golden Turtle is a symbol for longevity. *Wu* longevity practices involve incorporating the turtle's ability to periodically avoid the intake of food, instead finding nourishment through eating Qi with long, slow breaths. The Golden Turtle also represents the northern direction and the spiritual energy related to your kidneys— the very source of your life energy. Practicing Golden Turtle Mudra will help you strengthen your kidney function, enrich your life source, and promote longevity.

Visualization

Imagine your hands extend far away while you rotate your hands to gather the Universal Qi. Envision the Qi, like the light of the sun and moon, merging into your kidneys as your fingers point toward your kidneys.

Breathing

Take a deep breath while rotating your hands. On the exhale, sound the Mantras *Hai* 嗨 (pronounced "hi") and

Hei 嘿 (pronounced "hey") while pointing your fingers towards your kidneys. Practicing these two mantras will help you strengthen your kidney Qi (the root of your life energy) and may cure illnesses related to weak kidney Qi.

Benefit

In Chinese shamanism, we believe that when the Universe created Earth, it first gave birth to Water, subsequently creating the conditions for all life to come into existence. From the microcosm–macrocosm perspective, we can view both the Universe and the Earth as the model of our body. Just as the Universe first gave birth to Water (which in turn generated all life on Earth), the Water organ system in your body is considered to be the place where your life energy began. In Chinese shamanism and in Traditional Chinese Medicine, the kidney organ system is known as the Water organ system of your body, the place where your life first started and the root of your life source.

This practice will help you strengthen your kidney Qi and help you recognize the profound connection between your life energy and your kidneys. It is a great practice to help you recover from any kind of kidney related diseases (e.g. lower back pain, weak knees, tinnitus, weak bones, poor memory, and low sexual drive). As the place where your life energy is stored, strengthening your kidneys is also a traditional anti-aging method to keep you feeling young and healthy.

8

Wan Shen Chao Li

萬神朝禮

Cultivating Your Gratitude

萬神朝礼

庚寅孟冬　乾元子 书

Meaning

Wan 萬 means ten thousand, numerous, and countless. **Shen** 神 means stretch, brightening, marvelous, mystery, and spirit. **Chao** 朝 means gather, face, and pilgrim. **Li** 禮 means humble, humbleness, modest, courtesy, polite, ritual, and ceremony.

According to Chinese shamanism, everything, including each part of your body, has a spirit. The *Wanshen* 萬神 (Ten Thousand Spirits) of your body are formed by the essential Qi or vital energy of the associated parts of the body. The leader and core spirit of your body inhabits the *Niwangong* 泥丸宮 (Clay Pill Palace), which is located in or near the pineal gland of your brain. Among other things, the pineal gland secretes the hormone melatonin, which modulates your diurnal wake/sleep patterns and seasonal fluctuations of your body. Thus, one could say the pineal gland plays a vital role in keeping us in harmony with the rhythms of nature. In the context of your spiritual cultivation practices, your body will maintain wellness if all of your body spirits are connected to this leader spirit. In other words, you will live from a centered place of physical and mental balance if your whole body Qi is connected with *Niwangong*.

In the highest level of Qigong training, we achieve the *Lian Qi Hua Shen* 煉氣化神 state and transform our Qi into *Shen* or spirituality. To reach this stage, you must develop your humble nature and work to keep yourself centered. With dedication, you will be able to feel your Qi rising through your whole body and connecting with your brain and the Clay Pill Palace.

Wan Shen Chao Li is a way to help you cultivate your stableness, humbleness, and gratitude and to work towards the state of *Lian Qi Hua Shen*—feeling the spirits of your entire body celebrate peace in the Clay Pill Palace.

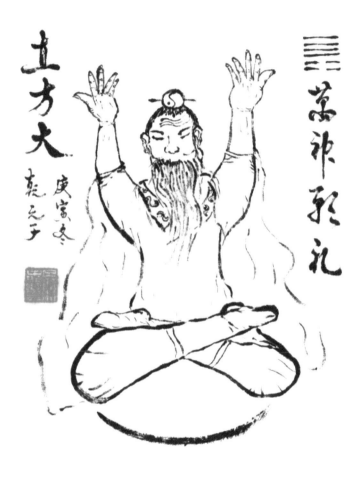

Figure 8. Cultivating Your Gratitude Posture

Movement

From the previous posture, rotate your cupped hands and raise them up alongside your body, towards your armpits. Keep spiraling your hands so that they pass by your ears with the fingers pointing upwards and palms facing backwards. Next, clench your teeth, lower your chin, curve your back, and bend your upper body and head down to the floor in front of you, or as low as you can. At the same time, gradually extend your arms down to the ground, ending with your forehead and hands (palms facing heaven) resting on the floor, with arms stretched out in front of you. This is **Chaoliyin** 朝禮印— Pilgrim Mudra (Figure 8). Practicing *Chaoliyin* will help you refine your modesty, strengthen your Yang Qi/life force, and nourish your brain.

Visualization

Imagine the Qi like sunlight ascending along your spine to reach the brain.

Breathing

Take a deep breath. While slowly exhaling, sound the Mantra **En** 嗯 through your clenched teeth as your curve your back and move towards the ground in front of you. *En* (pronounced "un") means grateful. Practicing this mantra will help uplift your spirit, rejuvenate your Yang Qi, and awaken your consciousness.

Benefit

This practice is a fantastic way to transform your *Jing* 精 (essence) to Qi 氣 (vital energy), and then your Qi to *Shen* 神 (spirit).

The fundamental principle of *Neidan* 內丹 (Internal Alchemy) or traditional Qigong practice is to refine and transform your *Jing*, the essential life source of your physical body, into Qi, the vital energy of your body, and then to transform your Qi into *Shen*, your spiritual bodies. We also call this practice *Lianye* 煉液, which means refine your liquid or water. This is because *Jing*, the essence of your physical body, is liquid. *Jing* is the origin of *Shen* (spirit).

As I discussed in the Meaning section of this chapter, the core spirit of your body is located in a high position in your body, in the pineal gland. *Jing*, however, acts like water and stays in a low position. The kidneys, situated well below your pineal gland, are considered to be the reservoirs of the *Jing*. How then, does water flow from the low position to the high position? Let us observe what happens in nature. We see that water on the earth (in the low position) reaches the sky (high position) every day through evaporation. Warm air near the Earth's surface (Earthly Qi) absorbs moisture in the form of invisible water vapor from bodies of water, moist ground, and from plants. This warm, moisture-laden air (Earthly Qi) then rises and forms clouds. When the water droplets in the clouds cool and condense, rain (Heavenly Qi) then falls back down to nourish the earth. This same process happens in your body—to transform the water (*Jing*) to steam or clouds (Qi), we must generate heat, or Yang energy. Through cultivation practices, we stoke our Inner Fire, and provide a pathway for our *Jing* to transform to Qi and ascend from the kidneys up through our body. After the Qi rises to nourish your *Shen*, you will physically feel your body producing more saliva in your mouth. Traditionally, we refer to our saliva as *GanLu* 甘露 (Sweet or Heavenly Dew). Like rain pouring down on the earth, as we swallow the Heavenly Dew down to our *Dantian*, we reunite our *Shen* with our physical body, nourishing each and every part of ourselves.

This practice will help you increase Yang energy and allow your Qi to flow freely in your *Du* 督 meridian, which is also known as the Governing meridian. The Governing meridian is located at the center of your back and runs (approximately) along your spine. As the name suggests, the Governing meridian governs or controls all the Yang energy of your entire body. In Chinese medicine, disease typically occurs when there is a stagnation, or disruption of flow, in the vital energy somewhere in the body. If there is no stagnation in your *Du* meridian and the Qi can flow freely within it, your Yang energy and Inner Fire will also flow freely, and you will be able to transform the *Jing* to Qi and Qi to *Shen*. Like ice transforming from solid to liquid to steam, disease-causing stagnation will melt away into a healthy state of free-flowing Qi. Regular practice of this form will ensure that your spirit reunites with all aspects of your body, nourishing each cell and providing an opportunity for you to experience many layers of healing.

9

Qi Chong Zi Xiao

炁沖紫霄

Uplifting Your Spirits

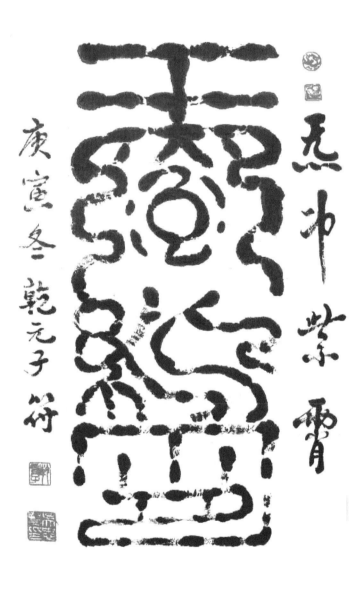

气冲紫霄

庚寅冬 范元子符

Meaning

Qi 炁 means vital energy or vital breath of nature. **Chong** 沖 means to mix, to infuse, to flush, to rise in the air, mingle, blend, charge, assault, and to collide with. **Zi** 紫 means purple, violet, and amethyst. **Xiao** 霄 means firmament, heaven, and the sky.

The written character Qi 炁 that I use here is different from the commonly written character Qi 氣, meaning vital energy. Qi 氣 is the basic element of the Universe. It is the same character found in the term Qigong 氣功. Most Chinese do not recognize the other written character (Qi 炁) that I am using as it only appears in old Chinese *Wu* 巫 (shamanic) or Daoist documents. The ancient character Qi 炁 is made with the upper radical *Wu* 无 and the bottom radical *Huo* 火. *Wu* means no, nothing, without, empty, emptiness, and the primordial state of nature or the Universe. *Huo* means fire. It is a symbol for mind, heart, spirit, desire, or anger in Chinese traditional spiritual cultivation. The distinction between the two characters can help us understand that the Qi 炁 referred to in ancient shamanic and Daoist texts is the refined or spiritualized Qi 氣 that is connected with the origin of your life and of the Dao. The lesser known Qi (炁) also means the vital breath of the Dao, or of nature. Once you can transform your vital energy Qi 氣 to spiritually refined Qi 炁, you reach a higher level in your Qigong practice and will feel your whole physical and spiritual body merging into a state of emptiness. In this purified state, your basic Qi 氣 is completely refined. You may feel as though your whole physical body is melting into warm sunlight. Your mind will be calm and relaxed without desire, anger, sadness, longing, worry, or excitement. Your consciousness, now fully awakened, will enable you to sense things that are happening within and outside your body.

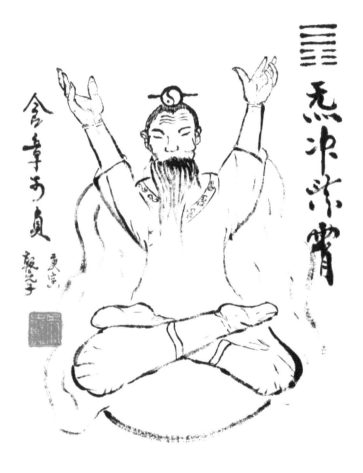

Figure 9. Uplifting Your Spirits Posture

In Daoist religion tradition, *Zixiao* 紫霄 is the name of the palace where the Lord Immortal *Laozi* 老子 (the author of the Daoist canon, the *Daodejing* 道德經) lives. It is often referred to as a sacred place where people live in freedom, peace, and harmony. With regards to your inner cultivation practice, it refers to the state of spiritual freedom of your mind. One of the purposes of our cultivation practice is to transcend your Qi (vital energy) into *Zixiao*, so that your mind will be in the state of spiritual freedom and harmony.

Qi Chong Zi Xiao training will help you transform your spirit and return to the Dao. In Chinese, this extremely high state of inner cultivation or Qigong practice is called *Lian Shen Huan Xu* 煉神還虛. It is a way to understand the state of oneness of the human being and nature. Through this practice, you will be able to fully awaken your consciousness and allow yourself to live from a place of spiritual autonomy.

Movement

From the previous posture, slowly straighten your back and neck and raise your upper body. At the same time, extend your arms above your head to form a V shape with your *Laogong* 勞宮 facing each other in the **Zixiaoyin** 紫霄印—Amethyst Celestial Mudra (Figure 9). Practicing this mudra will improve your ability to do remote healing and will help move you closer towards spiritual freedom.

Visualization

Imagine the Qi from your *Tianmen* 天門—Heavenly Gate (another name for the acupuncture point *Baihui* 百會 /GV20, which is located on the top of your head) and from your fingertips is penetrating Heaven to connect with the three heavenly treasures—the sun, moon, and stars. Feel your entire body dissolving into the heavenly treasures while you are making the Mantra *Weng*.

Breathing

Take a deep breath as you straighten your upper body. As you exhale, sound the Mantra **Weng** 嗡 (pronounced "wung") while you are holding your arms as a V shape above your head. The Mantra *Weng* means wise, and is voice of your spirit. Practicing this mantra will magnify your ability to emit your external Qi, which is a necessary skill when using remote Qi healing to help others.

Benefit

Regular practice of this form will help open your *Tianmen* (Heavenly Gate) and strengthen your spiritual energy. The acupuncture name for Heavenly Gate is *Baihui*, which literally means the gathering point of hundreds of Qi (vital energy) pathways. It is where all the meridians and channels of your body come together. Once you are able to open this point, the energy in all the meridians and channels of your whole body will be free flowing, and you will feel that your spirit is awake and free. The fundamental principle of health and healing in Chinese medicine maintains that healing occurs when the Qi is flowing freely in your meridians, channels, and entire body.

This practice will help you recover from suffering, whether it be born from a physical or an emotional illness. It also has powerful therapeutic functions, facilitating an experience of freedom within the physical and spiritual bodies, so that you may transcend into a highly cultivated or enlightened Qigong state.

10

Jin Guang Hui Zhao

金光回照

Brightening Your Body

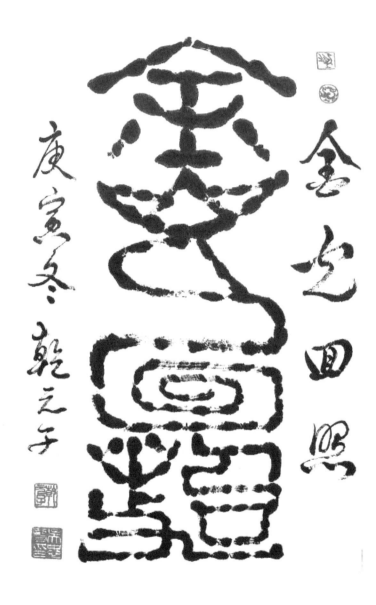

金光四照

庚寅冬 乾元子

Meaning

Jin 金 means metal, gold, and golden. **Guang** 光 means light, bright, and clear. **Hui** 回 means circle, go back, return, turn around, answer, and revolve. **Zhao** 照 means according to, shine, reflect, and illuminate.

In our inner cultivation practice, *Jinguang* 金光 (Golden Light) represents the high quality of the Qi related to your mind and spirit. There are Golden Lights surrounding your body that protect you and help you maintain your well-being when your heart/mind is pure and remains fully integrated within your body. The Golden Lights disappear from your body when you have a busy or uneasy mind. Where your mind goes, your Qi follows. If you can pay close attention to your body in your daily life, your Qi will be conserved in your body, which will allow you to transform it into Golden Light. If your mind is always busy, thinking about shopping, bills, your job, homework, tests, planning for the future, or ruminating on the past, your Qi is constantly out of your body. This will not only weaken your life energy, but will also inhibit you from being able to transform your Qi into Golden Light.

Make a habit of purifying your heart/mind in order to maintain the tranquil state which allows the Golden Lights to return to your body. In the highest level of your Qigong practice, you will be able to see your refined Qi as a golden brightening within your body. As a matter of fact, the ancient Chinese characters for spirit and brightening are the same! Ancient Chinese shamans considered brightening to be the spirit of nature and found that highly refined Qi, or cultivated spiritual energy, looked just like brightening within the body. You will live with an illuminated spirit and perception when you experience this for yourself. In this state, you will have no doubts about your life and you will know that you are

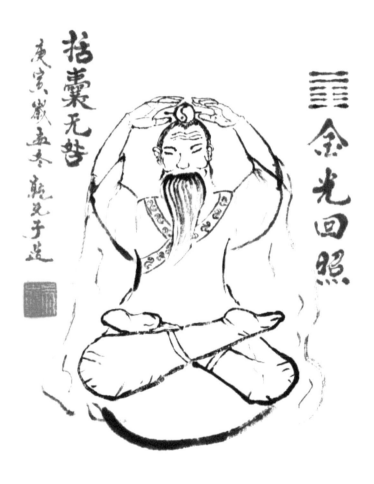

Figure 10. Brightening Your Body Posture

walking on your spiritual path. People around you, whether consciously or unconsciously, will enjoy your invisible radiant Qi field, your quiet serenity, and genuine wisdom.

Jin Guang Hui Zhao is a way to clear your mind, to purify your body in the deepest spiritual levels, to merge all aspects of yourself, and to experience the highest quality life.

Movement

From the previous posture, round your elbows so that your arms make a circle above your head. Your fingers point towards each other and your *Laogong* is directed at *Tianmen* (the top of your head) in *Jinguangyin* 金光印—Golden Light Mudra (Figure 10). Practicing this mudra will help you calm your mind, release your stress, and maintain a high level of well-being.

Visualization

Imagine bringing the Heavenly Qi in towards your body with your hands. Visualize the Qi as gold colored lights pouring into your body, from your hands through *Tianmen* (Heavenly Gate). Feel your whole body is soaking in the golden Qi field.

Breathing

Inhale a long, slow breath while turning your wrists. As you hold the mudra, keep your breathing slow, smooth, deep, and even. You can try holding the posture as long as you can.

Benefit

This practice will help you purify your body and mind by helping to release stagnation from your physical, emotional, and spiritual layers. It is one of the best ways to practice refining your Qi into the highest quality state, which will allow you to bring your Golden Lights back to your body. After several weeks of continuous practice, you will be able to feel the benefits of living with a clear, easy heart, and a body that is full of vitality.

11

Yue Lang Kun Lun
月朗昆侖

Awakening Your Inner Wisdom

月朗昆侖

庚寅冬 乾元子敬書

Meaning

Yue 月 means moon. *Lang* 朗 means clear, bright, and brighten. *Kun Lun* 昆侖 is the most sacred mountain in Chinese shamanic tradition, as it is the place where the Queen Mother of the West dwelt. We believe that the Queen Mother of the West was the first to have passed down the teachings of the shamanic and Daoist traditions. It is said that the Daoist teachings of Yellow Emperor, the ancient shaman king who is regarded as the founder of Chinese civilization (he lived about 5,000 years ago), and of Laozi, the author of *Daodejing* (the core Daoist text), came from her.

In Chinese inner cultivation practices, the moon symbolizes Yin energy whereas the sun symbolizes Yang energy. The luminescence of the moon (Yin) is simply a reflection of the brightness of the sun (Yang). In this spirit, during our Qigong practice we describe the different faces of the moon in terms of different stages of our Yang energy. We draw on the image of the new moon to represent the Yang energy at the very beginning of our practice, and that of the full moon to illustrate Yang energy reaching its peak level. We also describe different states of mind, consciousness, and wisdom in terms of various faces of the moon. A bright full moon, for example, is a picture of your clear, peaceful, and enlightened mind. In Chinese wisdom traditions, we refer to the brain, head, or spiritually realized states as *Kun Lun*. The clear full moon shining its light on *Kun Lun* Mountain is a depiction of the highest goal of our inner cultivation practice—to live our lives consciously and fully awakened.

Yue Lang Kun Lun is a way to look deep inside yourself, to awaken your consciousness, and to move through the world guided by your inner wisdom.

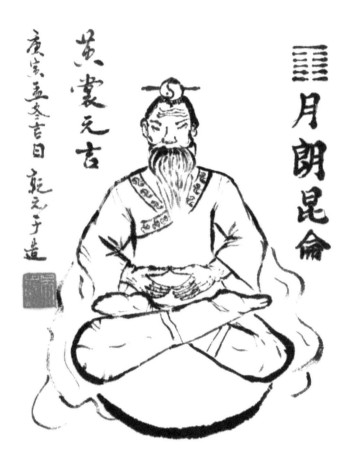

Figure 11. Awakening Your Inner Wisdom Posture

Movement

From the previous posture, with your palms facing earth, slowly bring your hands down your midline to your *Dantian* (lower belly). Then turn your palms towards your *Dantian* and have your thumbs and index fingers touch gently. Your *Laogong* on both hands will be facing your *Dantian* in **Yinguangyin** 銀光印—Silver Light Mudra (Figure 11). Practicing this mudra will help increase your Yin Qi, cultivate your gentleness, and reveal the source of great compassion for yourself and others.

Visualization

Imagine Qi, like a powerful waterfall, penetrating through your body when you bring your hands down to your *Dantian*. Imagine your hands covering the moon in your lower belly and that the light of the moon brightens your entire body as you hold the Silver Light Mudra.

Breathing

Take a deep breath and make the Mantra *Heng* 哼 (pronounced "hung") while exhaling and moving your hands down to the *Dantian*. *Heng* means sacrificial offering. Then, hold the mudra and regulate your breathing to be slow, smooth, deep, and even.

Benefit

Practicing this movement is a great way to open the *Ren Mai* 任脈 and to enhance your Yin Qi. *Ren Mai* is commonly translated as Conception Vessel in English. Running along the midline of the front aspect of your body, it is the meridian that rules Yin energy of your entire body. As Yin energy gives birth to Yang (life) energy, the *Ren Mai* also nourishes the Yang energy of your entire body. Your body will maintain a healthy state and a high level of wellness if your *Ren Mai* is open with the Qi flowing smoothly within it. This movement is beneficial for those who have Yin related health problems such as insomnia, high blood pressure, ADD (attention deficit disorder), ADHD (attention deficit hyperactivity disorder), migraines, anxiety, and poor stress management.

In order to have a harmonious body and a harmonious mind, and by extension, a harmonious society, it is necessary to have good quality Yin within. As Laozi states in his *Daodejing, wan wu fu Yin er bao Yang, chong Qi yi wei he* 萬物負陰而抱陽沖氣以為和 "When Yin embraces Yang, harmony is found."

12

Qing Jing Wu Wei

清靜無爲

Enjoying the Action-less

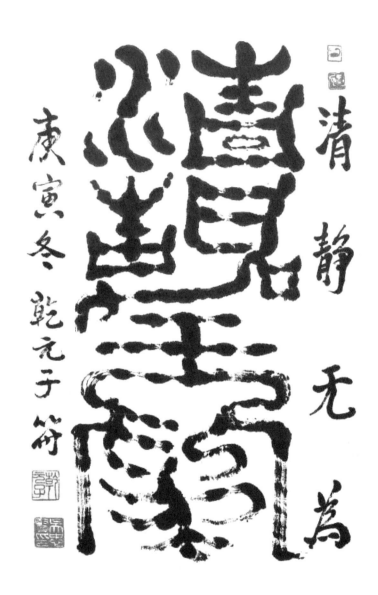

清静无为

康寅冬 乾元于都

Meaning

Originally, the meaning of **Qing** 清 is the clarity and purity of limpid water. In Chinese tradition, it is commonly used to describe that which is clear, clean, pure, bright, cool, fair, upright, peaceful, or elegant. *Jing* 靜 means still, motionless, silent, tranquil, peace, quiet, or stabilize. According to the Great Chinese Dictionary (from the Sichuan and Hubei Dictionary Publishing House), the original meaning of *Wu* 無 is dance or dancing. The purpose of Chinese *Wu* 巫 (shaman) dancing is to sublime your spirit into a state of emptiness, so that you can resonate with and understand the Dao, the great way of nature. However, at least a couple of thousand years ago, the Chinese character *Wu* 無 came to be used not for dancing, but for not, no, without, empty, nothing, nonexistence, emptiness, or nihility. *Wei* 爲 means do, act, make, study, plant, establish, think, believe, become, in order to, for, as, or action.

Qingjing 清靜 refers to a pure, tranquil state of the body and mind; it is the highest state of Qigong and other Chinese inner cultivation practices. As Laozi states in his *Qingjingjing* 清靜經 (*Tranquility Classics*), *ren neng chang qing jing tian di xi jie gui* 人能常清静天地悉皆歸 "Heaven and Earth will return to your body if you can remain in *Qingjing*." In order to reach this state of *Qingjing*, we have to embody *Wuwei* 無爲. Generally, we translate *Wuwei* as "action-less" in English. There is a common misconception in the West that the meaning of action-less is do nothing. *Wuwei* does not mean do nothing! In fact, *Wuwei* is an action. The action of *Wuwei* is exceedingly different from our regular daily activities. When we expend our energy through our general actions of daily living, we feel physically tired or/and mentally exhausted at the end of the day. However, if we turn our mind within and focus on our body, we will feel great and completely

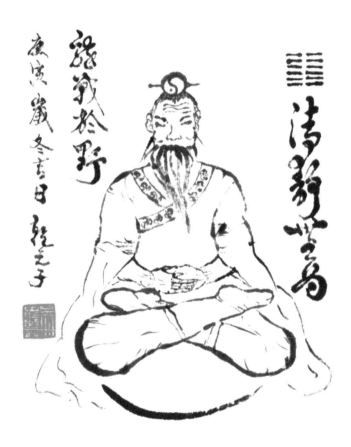

Figure 12. Enjoying the Action-less Posture

rejuvenated. The action of *Wuwei* involves allowing your *Shen* (spirit) to remain peaceful and calm within your body, regardless of your physical action. In the *Daodejing* 道德經, Laozi states *sheng ren wei wu wei zhi shi* 聖人爲無爲之事 "The sage conducts the *Wuwei* affairs." What are these *Wuwei* affairs? All traditional Chinese wisdom practices, such as playing Qin music, calligraphy, painting, Qigong, meditation, Taiji, and other internal martial arts can be considered *Wuwei* affairs if you truly master them.

Qing Jing Wu Wei is a way to conduct your *Wuwei* affairs, to merge into *Qingjing*, and to learn the art of living.

Movement

Bring your "tiger mouths" together over your *Dantian* to make **Taijiyin** 太極印 (*Taiji* Mudra). The tiger mouth is the curve between your thumb and index finger. Females will put their right hand inside the left, with the right palm touching the *Dantian*. The left thumb touches the right *Laogong* and the right thumb naturally rests on the *Hegu* 合谷 (LI4) point of the left hand. If you wiggle your thumb up and down, you will see a tendon sticking out on the back of your hand. The *Hegu* point is in on top of the muscle between your thumb and index finger, above that tendon. Males will make the same mudra, except with the left hand on the inside (Figure 12). Practicing *Taiji* Mudra will help you maintain a peaceful and tranquil state.

Visualization

Imagine gathering the Universal Qi into the *Dantian* and that there is a golden-red color sun in your *Dantian*. The sun brightens your whole body as you feel your body infusing with the lights of the sun.

Breathing

Allow your breath to become slow, smooth, deep, and even, just as you did in movement 1.

Function

Practicing this movement will help you preserve your Qi in the *Dantian*, enhance your life force, and maintain a sense of physical, mental, and spiritual well-being. Regular, dedicated practice of this form will allow you to experience the state of *Qingjing*—the state of oneness between human being and nature.

Quick Review Chart of the Wu 巫 (Chinese Shamanic) Cosmic Orbit Qigong

Movement	Sound (Mantra)	Mouth Position	Affected Area	Figure
Hands out in front	*Heng* (hung)	Closed	*Dantian* and Whole Body	1
Hands move to side	*Hu* (hoo)	Open	Spleen and Heart	2
Hands turn slightly behind	*Xu* (shhh)	Open	Five Organ Systems	3
Hands fold in and come straight out in front, facing outward	*Hong* (hoang)	Open	Heart	4, 5
Palms open, arms open to sides	*Ha* (ha)	Open	Lungs	6

Point fingers to lower back and motion down to kidneys	*Hai* (hi)/ *Hei* (hey)	Closed	Kidneys	7
Bring hands to the inside and extend upwards	*En* (un)	Closed	Up the Spine	8
Arms extend to heaven	*Weng* (wung)	Open	Top of Head (*Baihui*)	9
Bring hands and arms down to *Dantian* (lower belly)	*Heng* (hung)	Closed	3 *Dantian* and Whole Body	10, 11, 12

APPENDIX II

Quick Review of Movements

Please refer to the pages referenced in parenthesis for full information about the movement.

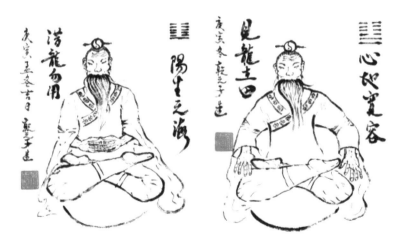

Figure 1 (page 25) *Figure 2* (page 35)

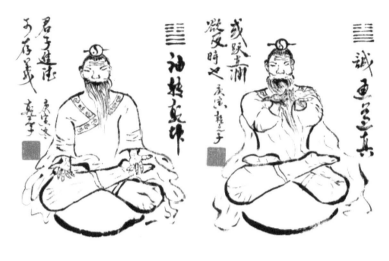

Figure 3 (page 41)   Figure 4 (page 49)

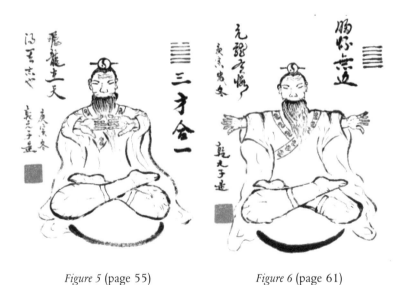

Figure 5 (page 55)   Figure 6 (page 61)

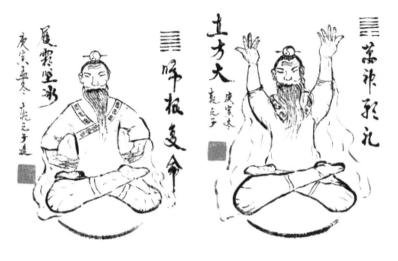

Figure 7 (page 67)   Figure 8 (page 73)

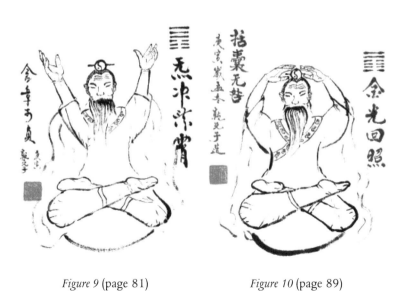

Figure 9 (page 81)   Figure 10 (page 89)

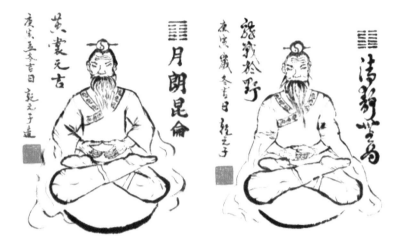

Figure 11 (page 95)   *Figure 12* (page 101)

About the Author

Master Zhongxian Wu was born on China's eastern shore in the city of Wenling in Zhejiang Province, where the sun's rays first touch the Chinese mainland. He began practicing Qigong and Taiji at an early age. Inspired by the immediate strengthening effects of this practice, Master Wu committed himself to the life-long pursuit of the ancient arts of internal cultivation. For over thirty years, he has devoted himself to the study of Qigong, martial arts, Chinese medicine, *Yijing* science, Chinese calligraphy, and ancient Chinese music, studying with some of the best teachers in these fields.

In China, Master Wu served as Director of the Shaanxi Province Association for Somatic Science and the Shaanxi Association for the Research of Daoist Nourishing Life Practices. In this capacity, he conducted many investigations into the clinical efficacy of Qigong and authored numerous works on the philosophical and historical foundations of China's ancient life sciences.

In 2001, Master Wu left his job as an aerospace engineer in Xi'an, China, to teach in the United States. For four years he served as Senior Instructor and Resident Expert of Qigong and Taiji in the Classical Chinese Medicine School of the National College of Natural Medicine (NCNM) in Portland, Oregon. In addition to his work at NCNM, Master Wu was a sub-investigator in a 2003 Qigong research program sponsored by the National Institute of Health (NIH).

Since he began teaching in 1988, Master Wu has instructed thousands of Qigong students, both eastern and western. Master Wu is committed to bringing the authentic teachings of Chinese ancient wisdom traditions such as Qigong, Taiji, martial arts, calligraphy, Chinese astrology, and *Yijing* science to his students. He synthesizes wisdom and experience for beginning and advanced practitioners, as well as for patients seeking healing, in his unique and professionally designed courses and workshops. He also offers a long-term Qigong training program which provides a strong foundation for the study of shamanic Qigong, internal alchemy, Taiji and Qi-healing skills (including classical Chinese energy techniques, Chinese calligraphy, medical Qigong, and martial arts applications). Please visit www.masterwu.net for further details about his teachings.

Master Wu has published eight books (five of which were written and published in China), and numerous articles on the philosophical and historical foundations of China's ancient life sciences, including the first the first Chinese Shamanic Qigong book in English, *Vital Breath of the Dao—Chinese Shamanic Tiger Qigong (Laohu Gong)*, also published by Singing Dragon.

Master Wu and his wife, Karin, currently reside in Virginia's Blue Ridge mountains where they founded Blue Willow Health Center (www.bluewillowhealthcenter.com).